COVID SCARIDY

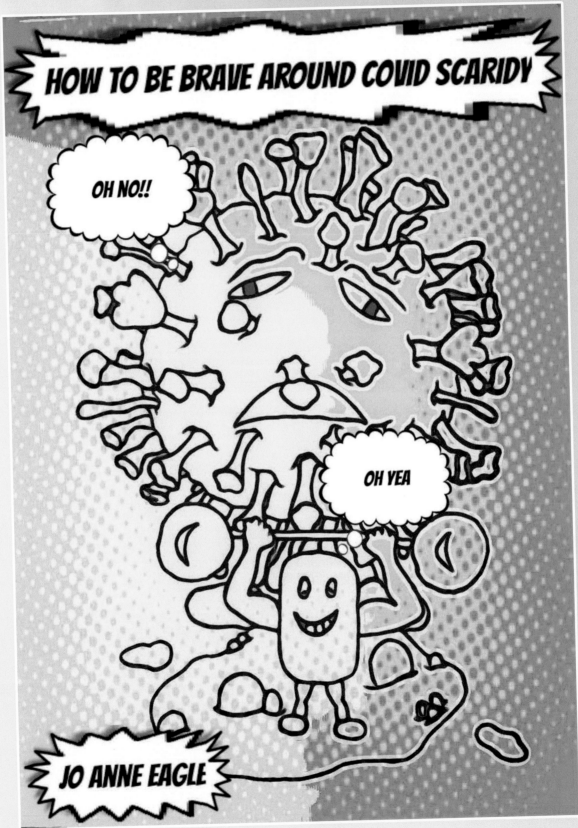

To order additional copies of this book, contact:
Xlibris
NZ TFN: 0800 008 756 (Toll Free inside the NZ)
NZ Local: 9-801 1905 (+64 9801 1905 from outside New Zealand)
www.xlibris.co.nz
Orders@Xlibris.co.nz

ISBN: 978-1-5434-9633-8 (sc)
ISBN: 978-1-5434-9632-1 (e)

Print information available on the last page.

Rev. date: 06/05/2020

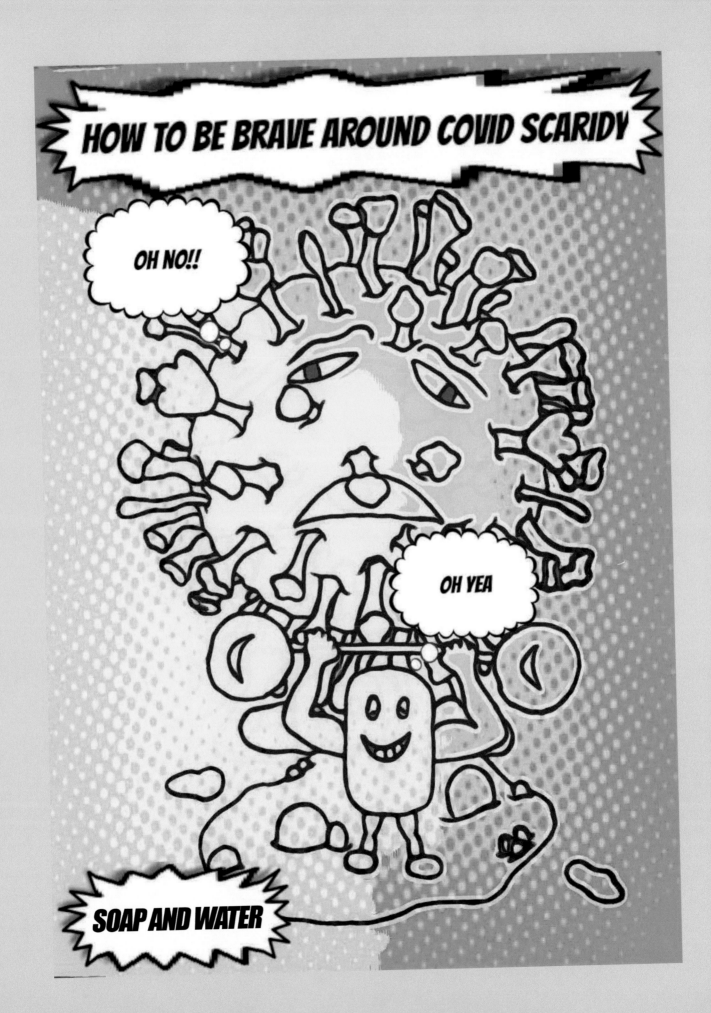

COLOUR ME IN

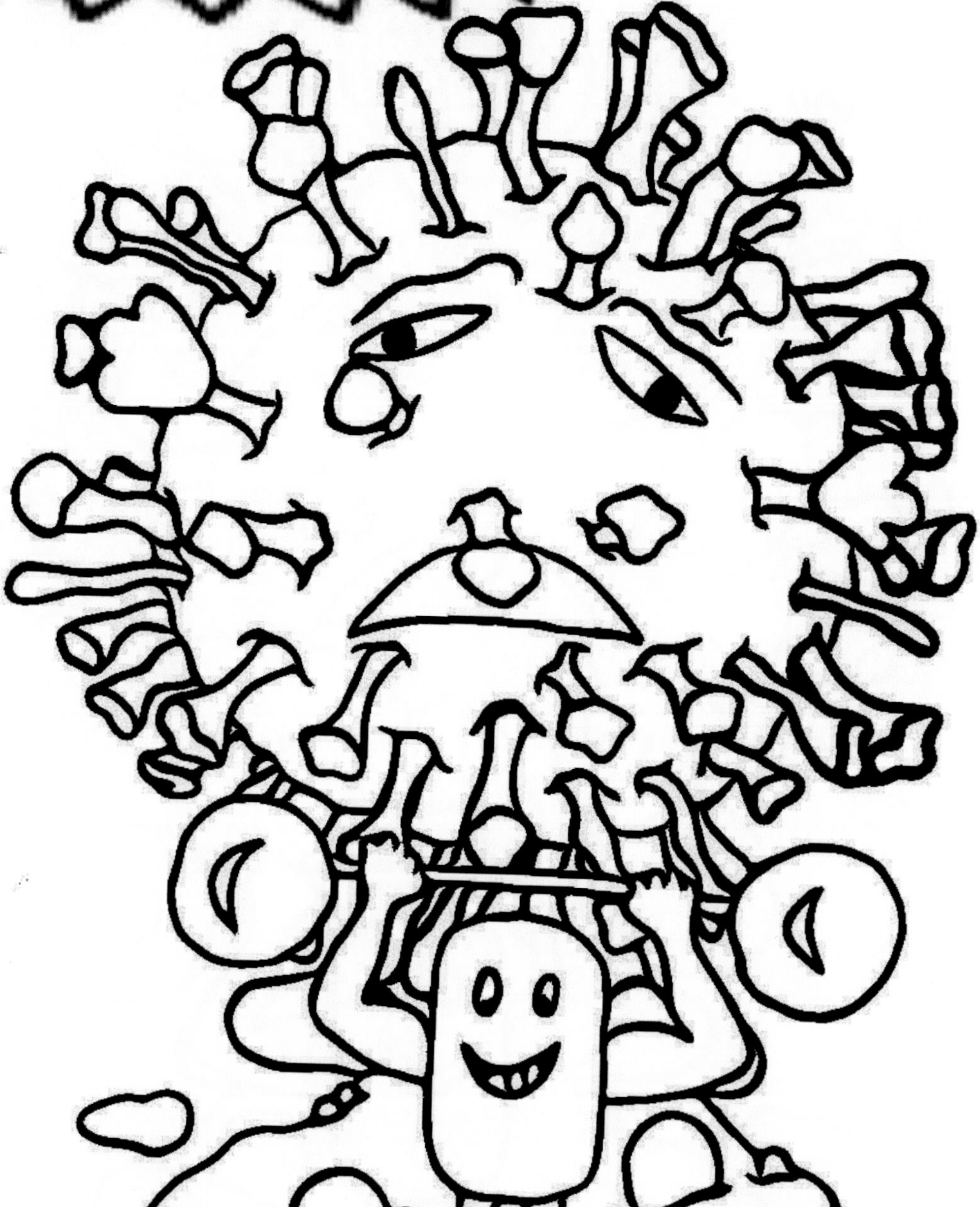

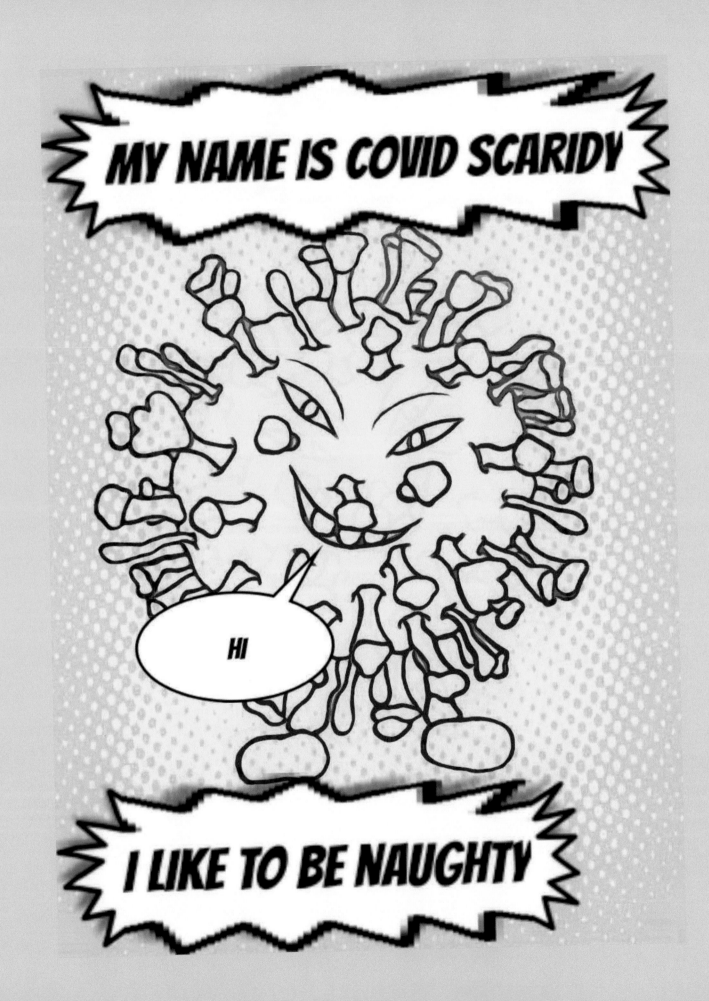

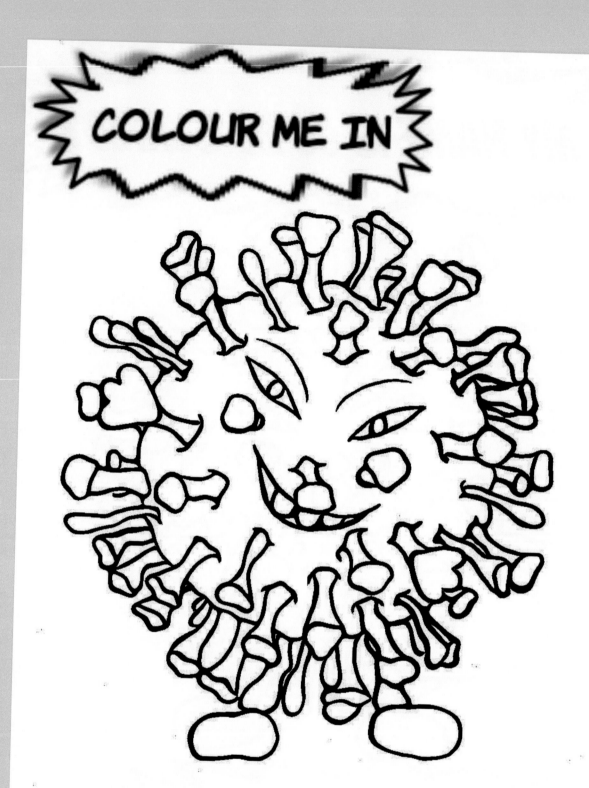

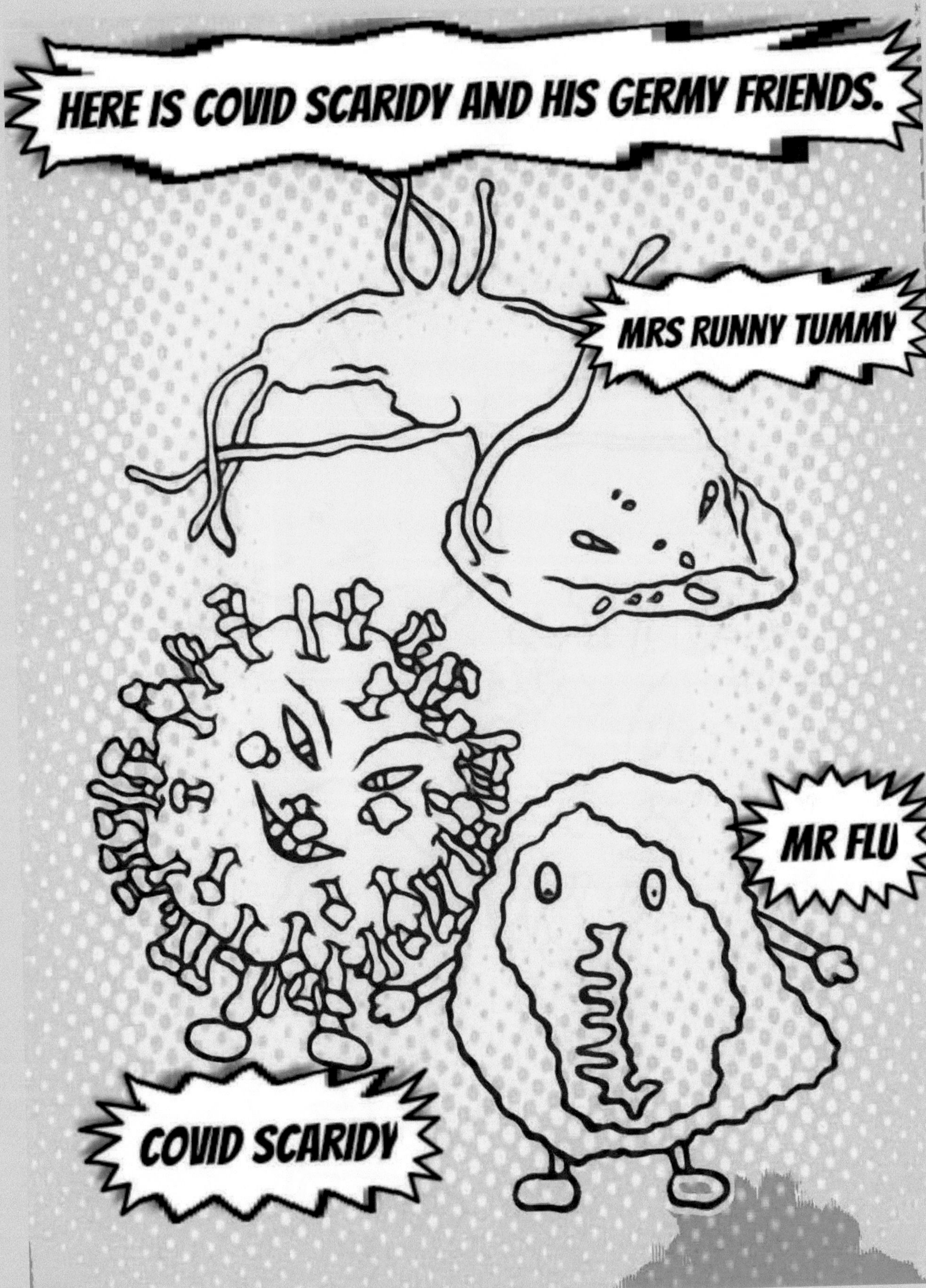
HERE IS COVID SCARIDY AND HIS GERMY FRIENDS.
MRS RUNNY TUMMY
MR FLU
COVID SCARIDY

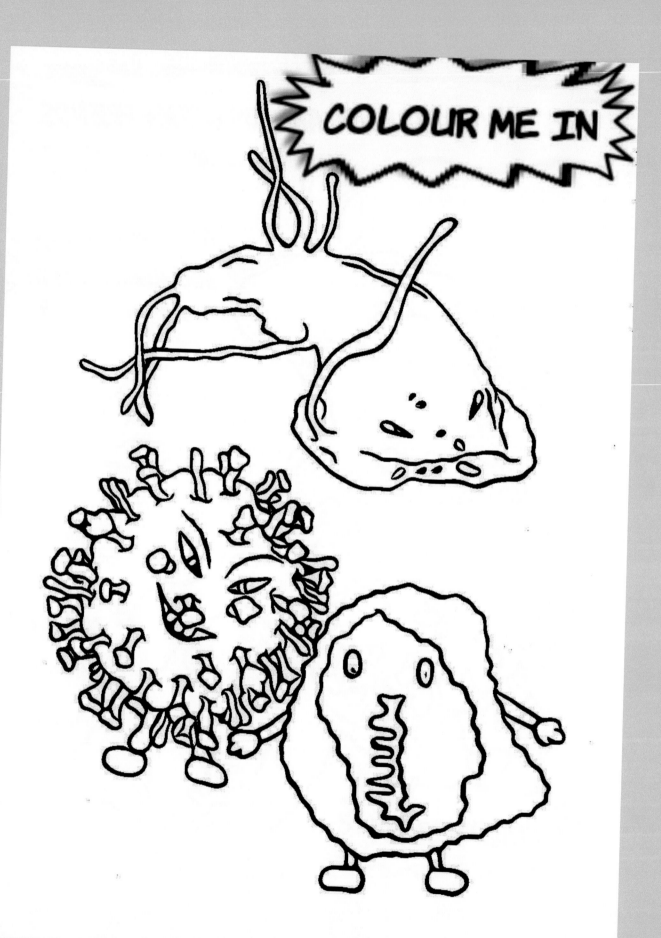

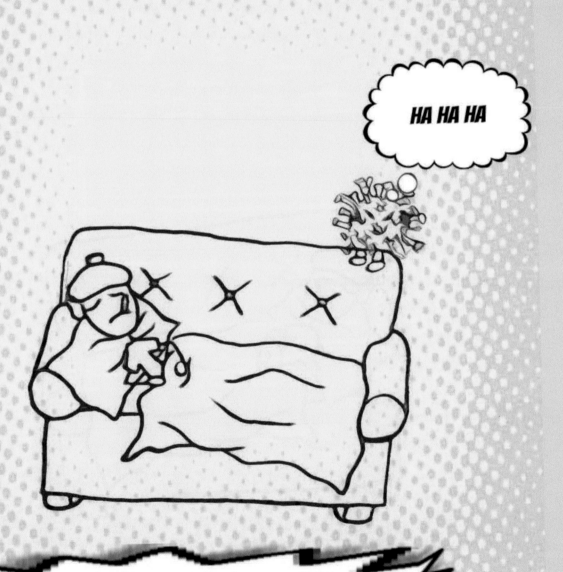

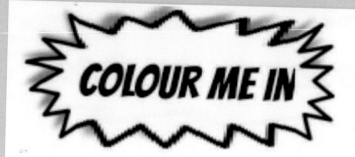

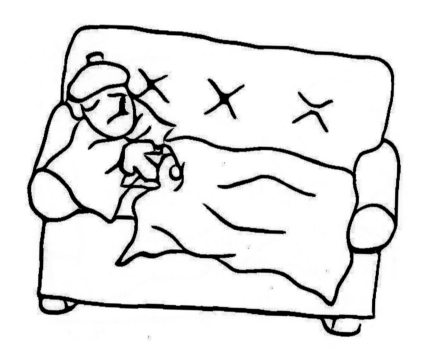

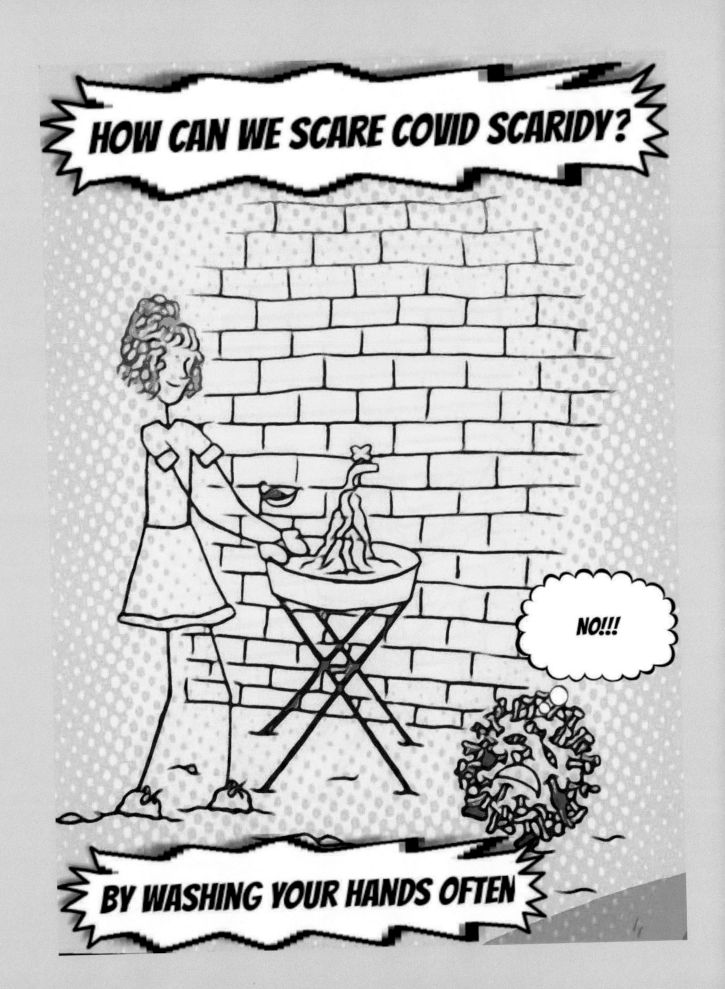

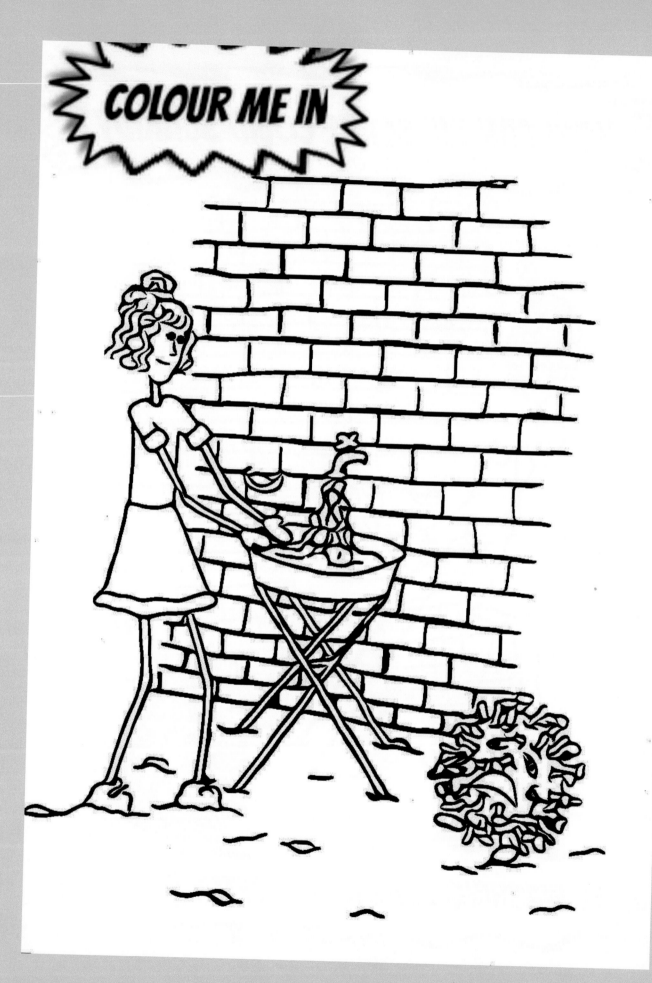

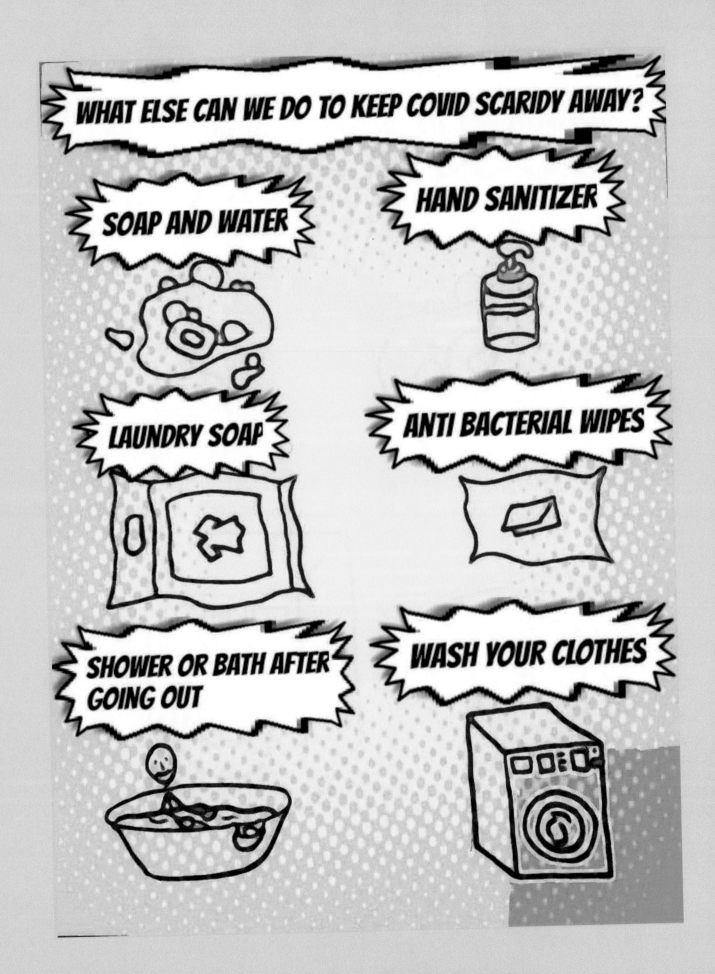

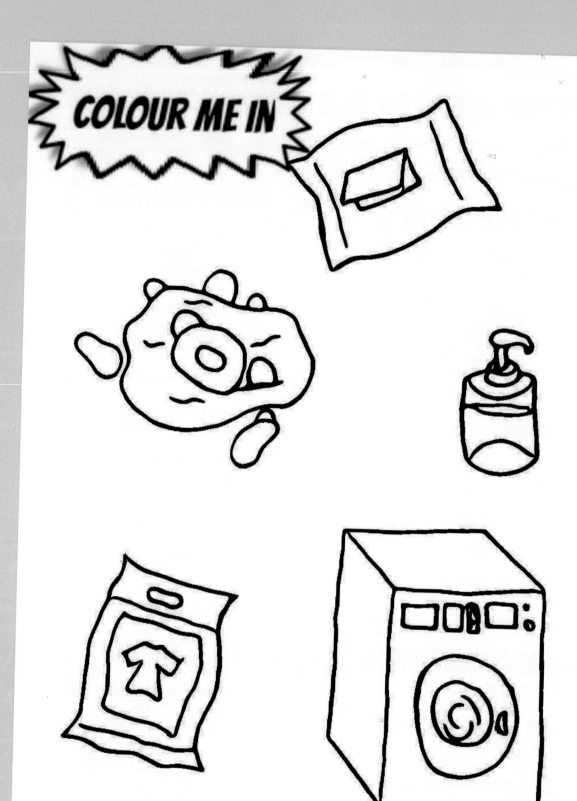

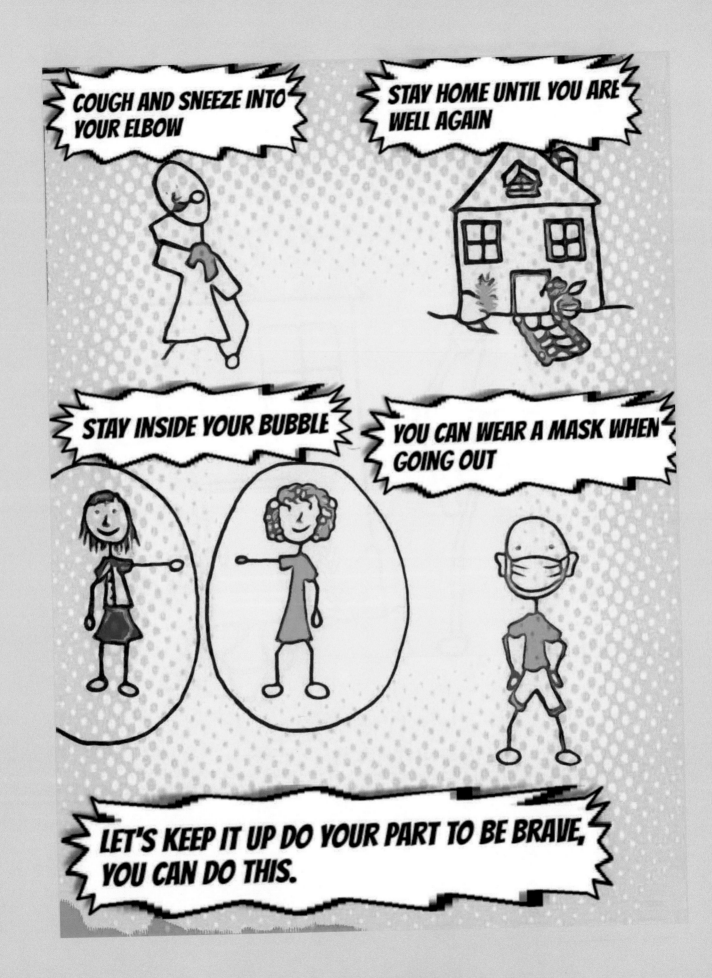

COLOUR ME IN

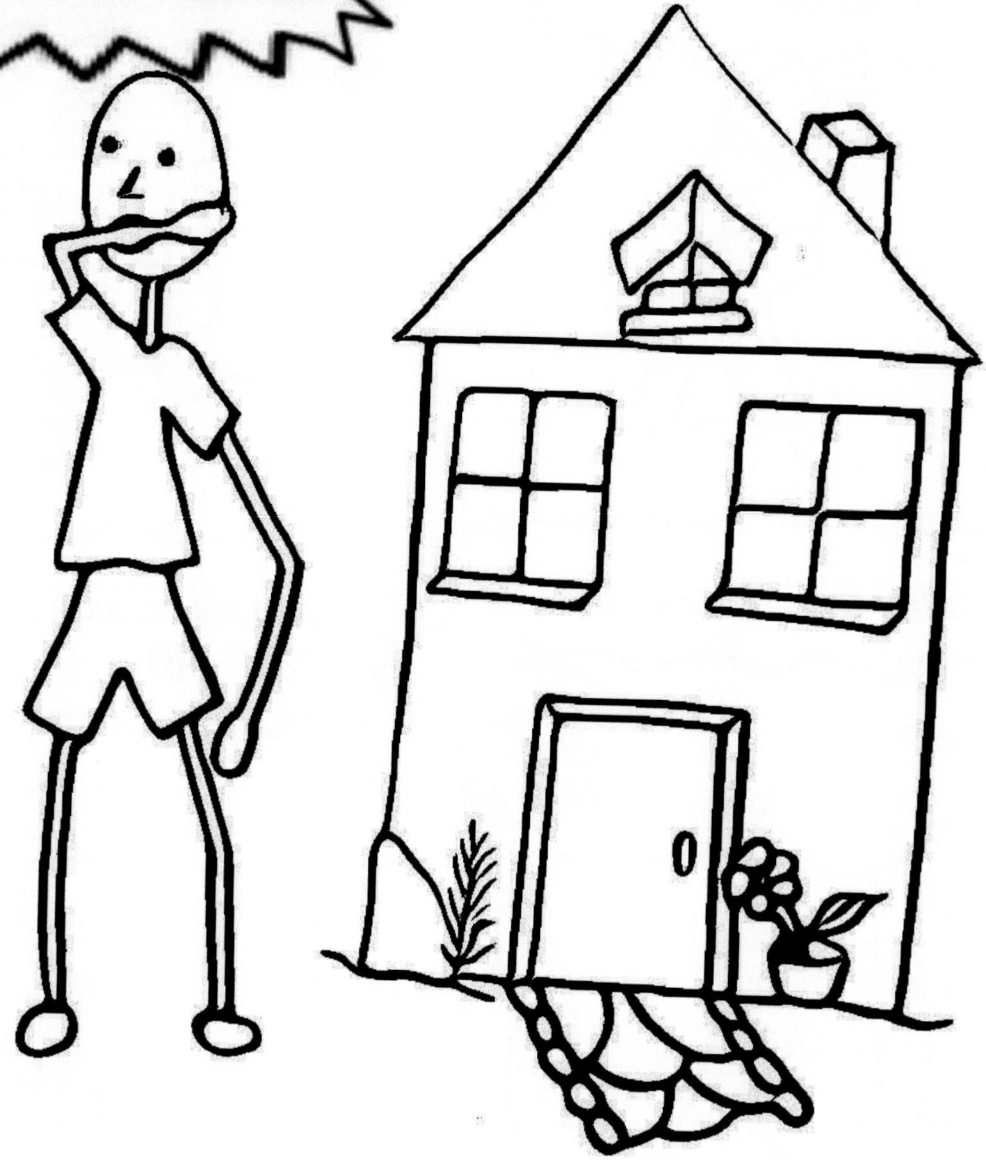

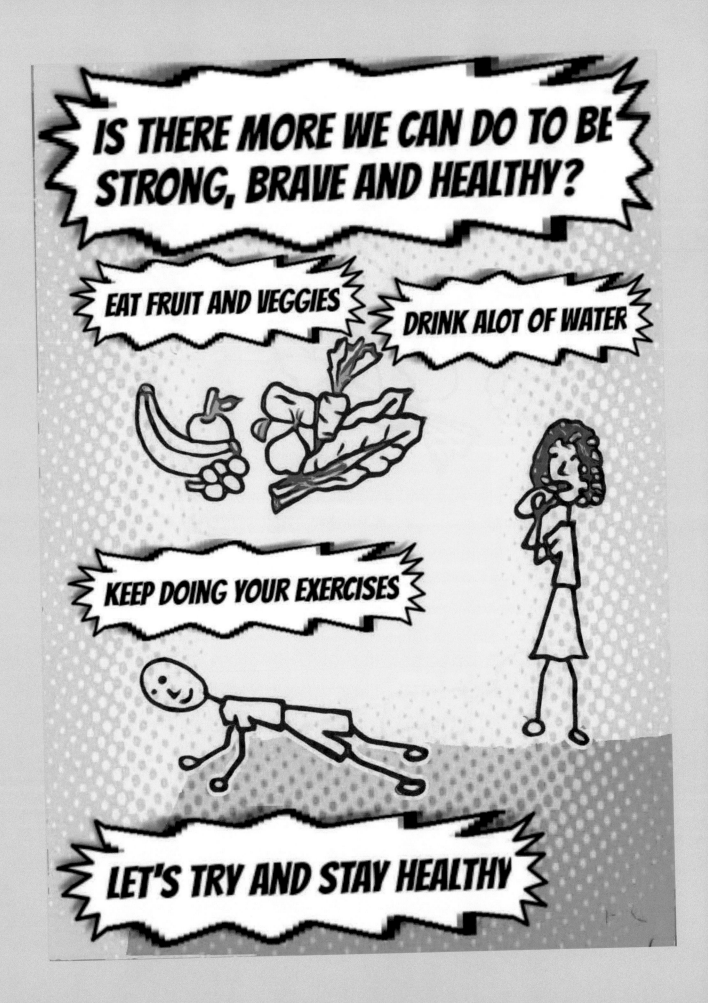

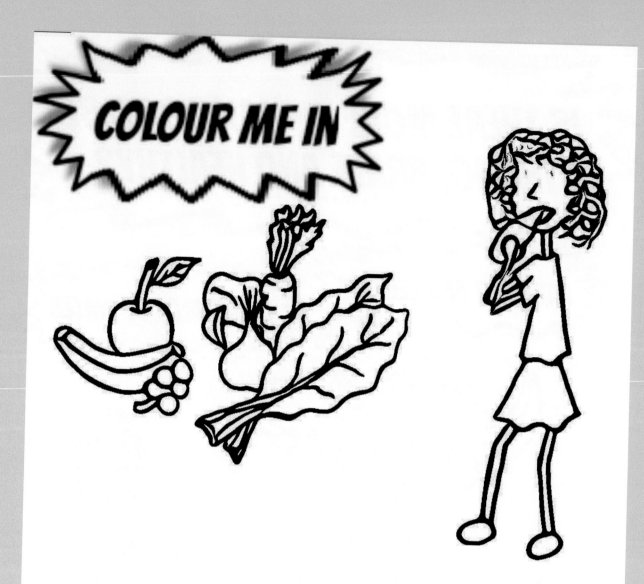

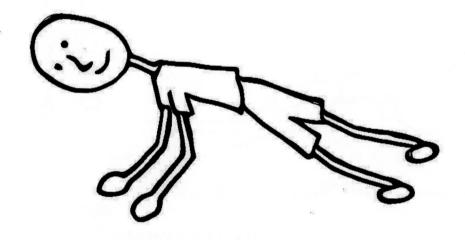

COVID SCARIDY DON'T LIKE CLEAN HANDS, OR HEALTHY CHILDREN.

HEALTHY CHILD

CLEAN HANDS

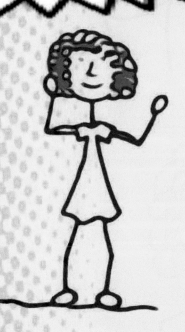

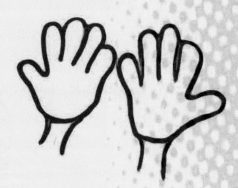

YAY!!! THAT'S GOOD TO KNOW DON'T YOU THINK SO?

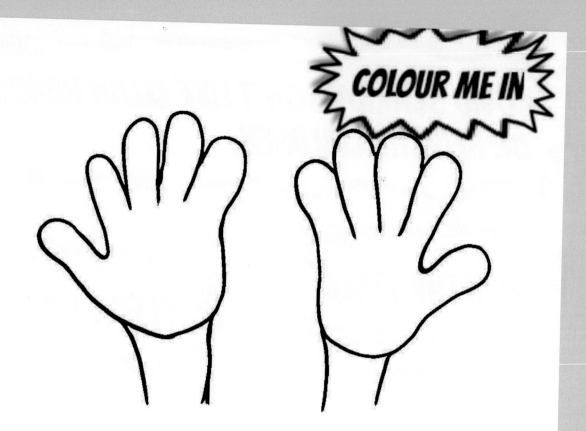

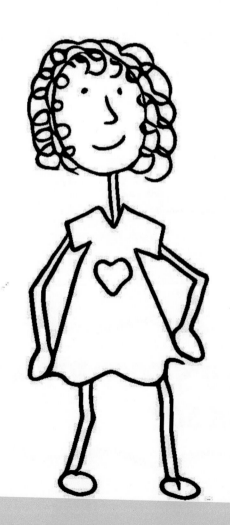

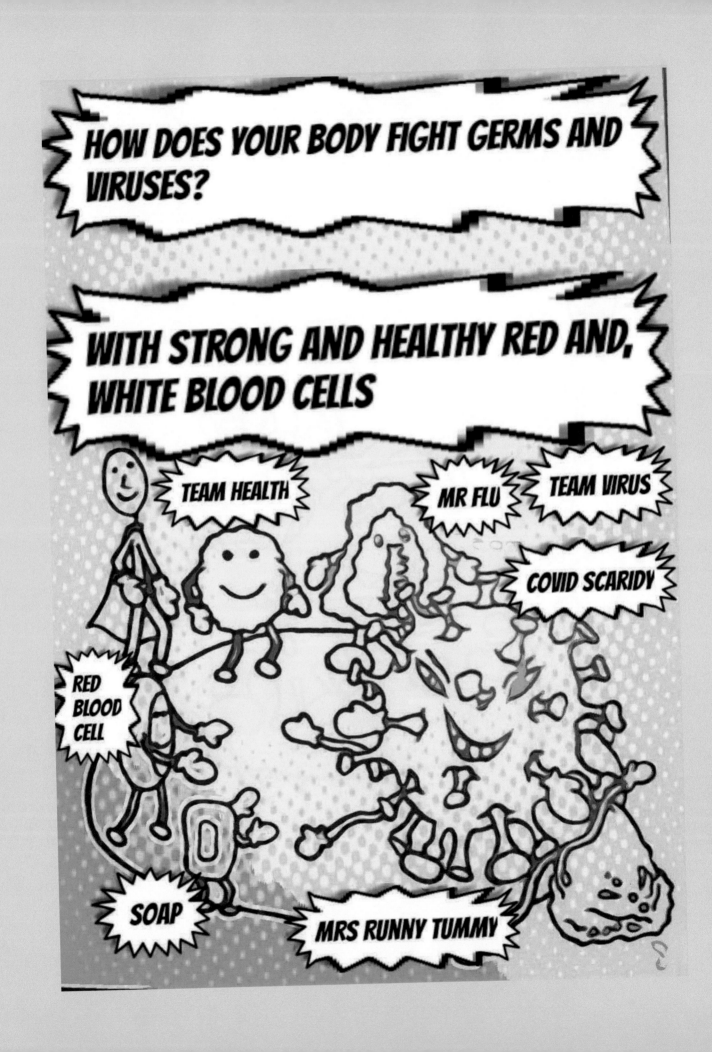

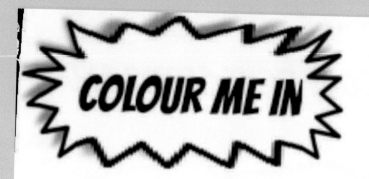

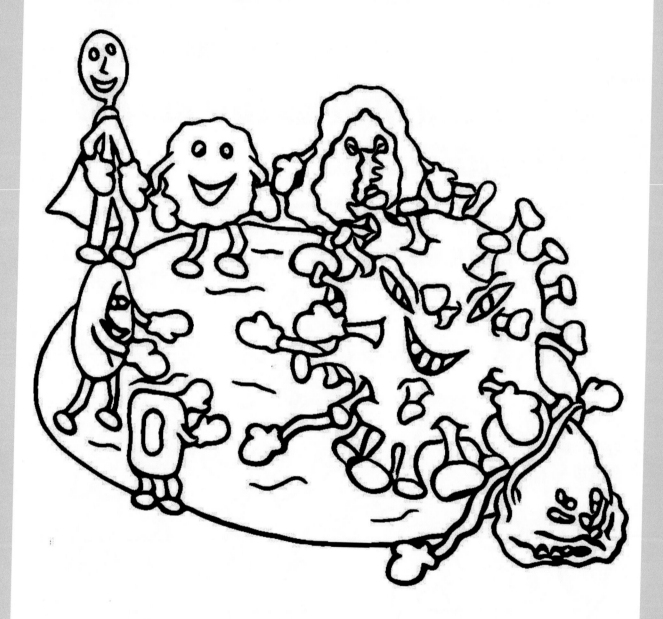

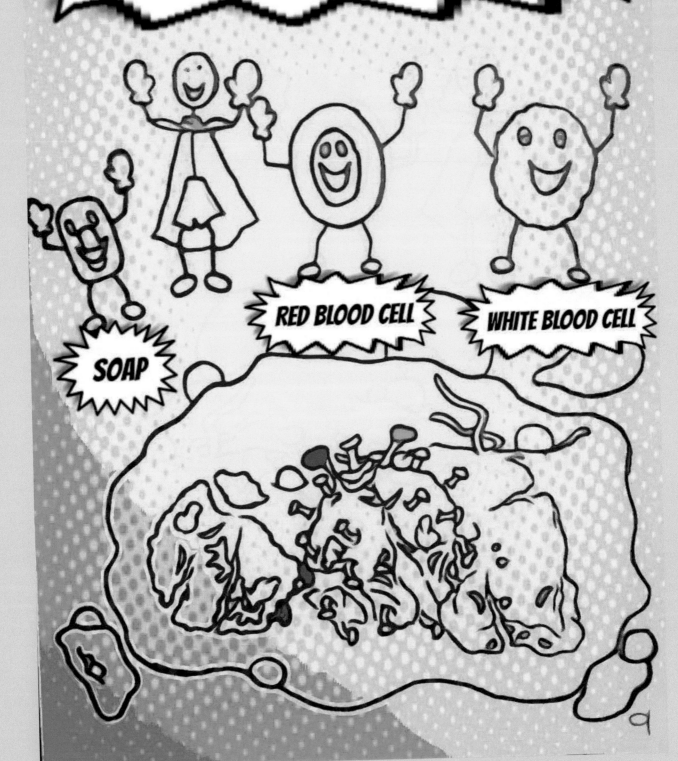

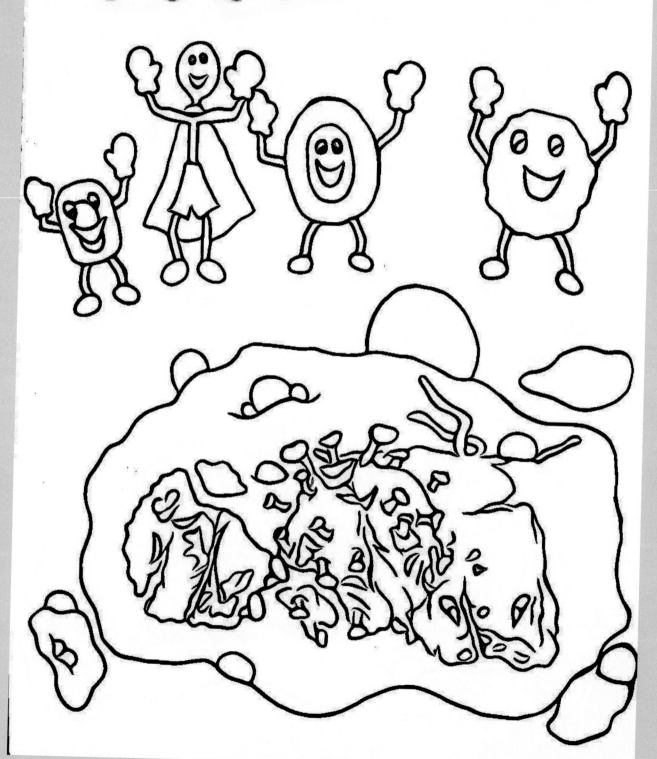

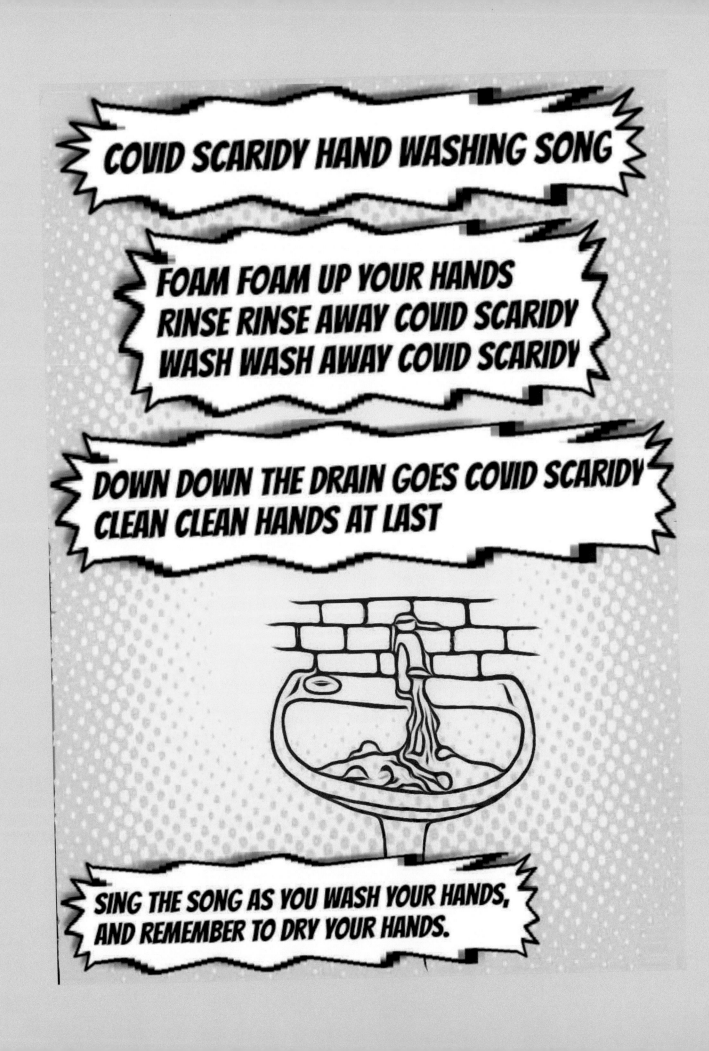

Printed in the United States
By Bookmasters